Childhood Cancer

All about cancer and how to overcome childhood cancer

By

Georgia G. Walker

TABLE OF CONTENT

Introduction

Cancer occurs when cells develop uncontrollably and spread.

Cancer can start at any place in the trillion-cell human body.

Human cells divide to create new cells as needed.

New cells replace old or injured ones.

When this ordered process fails, aberrant or damaged cells proliferate and multiply.

These cells can create cancers.

Cancerous or non-cancerous tumors (benign).

Cancerous tumors infect neighboring tissues and can generate new tumors elsewhere in the body (a process called metastasis).

Malignant tumors are cancerous.

Leukemias, for example, rarely form solid tumors.

Benign tumors don't spread.

Benign tumors rarely return, although malignant ones sometimes do.

Benign tumors can grow huge.

Benign brain tumors can be life-threatening.

Cancer vs. Normal Cells

Cancer cells differ significantly from normal cells.

Cancer cells develop without signals.

Normal cells only proliferate with such impulses.

• disregard cell division and death signals (a process known as programmed cell death or apoptosis).

• spread to other body parts.

Most normal cells do not migrate and cease growing when they encounter other cells.

• direct blood vessels to malignancies.

These blood channels feed and clean malignancies.

• evade the immune system.

The immune system destroys damaged or diseased cells.

• fool the immune system into supporting cancer growth.

Some cancer cells persuade immune cells to protect the tumor.

• have chromosomal duplications and deletions.

Cancer cells have double the chromosomes.

• use different nutrients.

Some cancer cells use nutrients differently to generate energy.

Cancer cells develop faster.

Cancer cells often need these aberrant characteristics to survive.

Researchers have used this to build cancer cell-targeted treatments.

Some cancer treatments starve tumors.

What Causes Cancer?

ENLARGE

Gene alterations cause cancer.

Chromosomes contain genes.

Changes to genes that regulate cell growth and division cause cancer.

Genetic alterations that cause cancer can result from cell division errors, DNA damage from environmental factors like tobacco smoke and UV radiation, or inheritance from our parents.

Before cancer develops, the body destroys damaged DNA cells.

Aging reduces the body's ability to do so.

This contributes to later-life cancer risk.

Each malignancy has unique genetic alterations.

Changes will occur as cancer grows.

Different tumor cells may have different genetic alterations.

Cancer Basics

Cancer cells can leave the primary tumor and move via the blood or lymph system to produce new tumors.

Metastasis.

Uncontrolled cell division and tissue spread cause cancer.

DNA alterations cause cancer.
Genes include most cancer-causing DNA alterations.
Genetic alterations are these.

DNA changes can make normal cell growth genes oncogenes.
Oncogenes, which cannot be turned off, promote uncontrolled cell growth.
Tumor suppressor genes inhibit cell proliferation in normal cells, preventing cancer.
Inactivating tumor suppressor genes can cause uncontrolled cell proliferation and malignancy.

The tumor microenvironment—immune cells, fibroblasts, molecules, and blood vessels—surrounds cancer cells.
Cancer cells can alter the microenvironment, affecting growth and dissemination.

Immune cells target cancer cells.
Some cancer cells can evade detection or attack.
Some cancer treatments help the immune system detect and eliminate cancer cells.

Each malignancy has unique genetic alterations.
Certain genetic variations may affect how cancer responds to treatment.

Cancer-causing genetic alterations might be inherited or environmental.
Cell division faults generate genetic alterations.

Cancer-causing genetic alterations usually build slowly as a person ages, increasing their cancer risk later in life.
Cancer cells can leave the primary tumor and move via the blood or lymph system to produce new tumors.
Metastasis.

Uncontrolled cell division and tissue spread cause cancer.

DNA alterations cause cancer.
Genes include most cancer-causing DNA alterations.
Genetic alterations are these.

DNA changes can make normal cell growth genes oncogenes.
Oncogenes, which cannot be turned off, promote uncontrolled cell growth.

Tumor suppressor genes inhibit cell proliferation in normal cells, preventing cancer.
Inactivating tumor suppressor genes can cause uncontrolled cell proliferation and malignancy.

The tumor microenvironment—immune cells, fibroblasts, molecules, and blood vessels—surrounds cancer cells. Cancer cells can alter the microenvironment, affecting growth and dissemination.

Immune cells target cancer cells.
Some cancer cells can evade detection or attack.
Some cancer treatments help the immune system detect and eliminate cancer cells.

Each malignancy has unique genetic alterations.
Certain genetic variations may affect how cancer responds to treatment.

Cancer-causing genetic alterations might be inherited or environmental.
Cell division faults generate genetic alterations.

Cancer-causing genetic alterations usually build slowly over time, increasing cancer risk later in life.

Cancer cells can leave the primary tumor and move via the blood or lymph system to produce new tumors. Metastasis.

Cancer Genes

Cancer-causing genetic alterations affect proto-oncogenes, tumor suppressors, and DNA repair genes. Cancer "drivers" are these alterations.

Normal cell division requires proto-oncogenes. These genes can become cancer-causing oncogenes when mutated or overactive, allowing cells to grow and survive when they shouldn't.

Tumor suppressor genes regulate cell growth and division.

Tumor suppressor gene mutations can cause uncontrolled cell division.

DNA repair genes repair DNA.

Mutations in these genes cause other gene mutations and chromosome alterations like duplications and deletions. These mutations may cause cancer.

As scientists learn more about cancer's molecular changes, they've found that some mutations occur in many cancers.

Many cancer treatments exist now.

Anyone with a targeted mutant cancer can use some of these treatments.

Chapter 1

The factors that lead to cancer in children

It is distressing to get a cancer diagnosis at any age, but it is more painful when the patient is a child. It is normal to have many questions, like, "Who should treat my child?" Will my child get well? What does this entail for our home and our loved ones? Although not every question is answered, the information and resources provided on this page are a good place to begin understanding the fundamentals of childhood cancer.

Some forms of cancer in children have been connected to certain environmental conditions, like the possibility of being exposed to radiation. Some research has also suggested that some parental exposures (like smoking, for example) can raise a child's risk of developing certain types of cancer; however, additional research is required to investigate these potential linkages. To this day, most malignancies diagnosed in children have not been demonstrated to have environmental roots.

Researchers have achieved considerable advancements in this field in recent years. Their understanding of how particular mutations in the DNA found inside our cells can lead to the development of cancer. DNA is the molecule composed of our genes, which are responsible for practically all of the activities in our cells. Because our DNA comes from our parents, we often take after the appearance of our parents. However, our DNA is responsible for far more than just our appearance. In addition, it affects the likelihood that we may get certain diseases, including some types of cancer.

The timing of when our cells grow, divide, and eventually die is determined by certain genes.

• Oncogenes are specific gene that helps cells grow, increase, or maintain their viability.

• Genes that inhibit the process of cell division, correct errors in the DNA of a cell, or trigger the death of cells at the appropriate time are referred to as tumour suppressor genes.

Cancers can be caused by alterations in the DNA that either continue to keep oncogenes turned on or turn off genes that prevent tumour growth.

Some children inherit alterations (mutations) in their DNA from one or both of their parents, putting them at an increased risk of developing certain types of cancer. These alterations are present in every cell of the child's body and can frequently be tested for in the DNA of blood cells or other body cells. Additionally, they are present in every organ of the child's body. Some of these DNA mutations are solely associated with an increased risk of cancer. Still, others can generate syndromes that include cancer and other health or developmental issues. However, most children's malignancies are not brought on by inherited mutations in DNA. They are the product of modifications to the child's DNA in the early stages of their development, sometimes even before birth. A cell must copy its DNA whenever it undergoes cell division into two new cells. Errors are inevitable in this process since it is not foolproof, particularly when the cells increase rapidly. An acquired mutation is the name of the gene change that can occur at any point in a person's life. Cancer cells are the only cells in the body that have acquired mutations; hence these changes cannot be passed on to the person's offspring.

There are occasions when the reasons for the changes in genes that particular adult malignancies undergo are known (such as cancer-causing chemicals in cigarette smoke). However, the factors that lead to DNA alterations in most children's malignancies are not well understood. Some could have external origins, such as exposure to radiation, while others could have internal causes that have not yet been identified. But it's quite likely that many of them are the consequence of random events, which can take place occasionally within a cell but don't have an external origin.

Important information regarding the following:

• It is estimated that 400 000 children and adolescents between the ages of 0 and 19 are diagnosed with cancer each year.

• Leukemia, brain malignancies, lymphomas, and solid tumours such as neuroblastoma and Wilms tumours are the most prevalent forms of juvenile cancer. Other types of childhood cancer include Hodgkin lymphoma and neuroblastoma.

• More than eighty per cent of children diagnosed with cancer can be cured in high-income nations thanks to the widespread availability of comprehensive treatment options. Less than thirty percent of people are healed in low- and middle-income countries (LMICs).

•Most cases of cancer diagnosed in children cannot be avoided or detected through screening.

•Most cancers that occur in children can be cured with over-the-counter medications and several other forms of treatment, such as surgery and radiation therapy. Treating juvenile cancer can be financially viable for families of all economic levels.

• In low- and middle-income countries (LMICs), avoidable fatalities from childhood cancers are caused by a lack of diagnosis, a misdiagnosis or a delayed diagnosis, impediments to receiving care, abandonment of treatment, death from toxicity, and relapse.

Comparatively, only 29% of low-income nations and 96% of high-income countries indicate that cancer treatments are generally available to their populations.

• Data systems on childhood cancer are necessary to propel ongoing improvements in the standard of care and inform public policy choices.

Cancer can strike individuals of any age and can spread to any organ or tissue in the body. It begins with a change in the genetic material of a single cell, which then multiplies and forms a mass (also known as a tumour), which, if untreated, can spread to other regions of the body, causing damage and ultimately leading to death. In contrast to malignancies that affect adults, the great majority of cancers that affect children have no identifiable root cause. A significant amount of study has been put into figure out what causes pediatric cancer. Still, the reality is that only a very small percentage of childhood cancers are caused by variables related to the environment or the child's lifestyle. Cancer prevention efforts directed at children should center on encouraging behaviors that protect them from contracting cancers that can be prevented when they are an adult.

Several persistent infections, including HIV, Epstein-Barr virus, and malaria, are recognized as carcinogens in children and adolescents. They are especially important for low- and middle-income countries. It is important to get vaccinated (against hepatitis B to help prevent liver cancer and against human papillomavirus to help prevent cervical cancer) and to pursue other methods, such as early detection and treatment of chronic infections that can lead to cancer. Other infections can increase a child's risk of developing cancer as an adult, so it is important to get vaccinated. Other infections can increase a child's risk of developing cancer as an adult.

According to the most recent statistics available, around 10% of all children diagnosed with cancer have a hereditary propensity for the disease. Additional research is required to discover the factors contributing to cancer development in youngsters.

The diagnosis of cancer in a youngster is extremely upsetting. There are likely dozens of concerns parents have regarding their child's health, treatment, and future, one of which is expected to be: how did my child develop cancer?

It is necessary to have a working knowledge of cancer to comprehend the factors that bring about the disease in youngsters. The mutation or change in DNA within a cell is the root cause of all malignancies, even those that develop in adulthood. In most cases, the body eliminates the new partition before it can do any harm.

On the other hand, when a person has cancer, the altered cell continues to expand and divide, producing new cells. Cancer cells can multiply and spread considerably more rapidly than healthy cells. They have the potential to spread throughout the body, which can lead to the development of tumours.

It is yet unknown what causes the majority of juvenile malignancies. A hereditary mutation is responsible for approximately 5 percent of all cases of cancer found in youngsters (a genetic mutation that can be passed from parents to their children).

It is believed that the majority of cancers that occur in children, much like those in adults, are the consequence of gene abnormalities. These mutations cause uncontrolled cell proliferation, which finally results in cancer. When found in adults, these gene changes reflect the cumulative effects of ageing and long-term exposure to drugs that can cause cancer. However, determining childhood cancer's possible environmental causes has proven difficult. This results in part from the fact that cancer in children is uncommon, and partly due to the fact that it is difficult to ascertain what children may have been exposed to during the early stages of their development.

Cancer is more likely to respond favorably to effective treatment and result in a larger possibility of survival when it is detected at an earlier stage. Early detection also results in less suffering and, frequently, lower costs and less rigorous therapy. It is feasible to make substantial advancements in the lives of children who have cancer by discovering the disease at an early stage and preventing delays in treatment. When treating children who have cancer, it is vital to have an accurate diagnosis because each type of cancer requires a unique treatment program that may include chemotherapy, radiation therapy, and surgery.

The ability to access prompt treatment is one of the three components that make up early diagnosis. The first component is the awareness of symptoms by families and primary care providers. The second component is an accurate and timely clinical evaluation, diagnosis, and staging (determining the extent to which cancer has spread).

Early detection is important in every context and has been shown to enhance survival rates for a variety of malignancies. Programs to encourage early and accurate diagnosis have been successfully implemented in countries with a wide range of income levels. These programs are frequently the result of a collaborative effort between governments, civil society organizations, and nongovernmental organizations, with parent organizations playing an essential role. Fever, severe and persistent headaches, bone pain, and weight loss are some of the warning symptoms that are connected with childhood cancer. These symptoms can be noticed by families as well as by primary healthcare providers who have received the appropriate training.

In most cases, screening tests for children's malignancies are not beneficial. It is possible to take into consideration high-risk populations in particular instances. If a mutation or disease is found in the family of a child who has been diagnosed with retinoblastoma, then genetic counselling can be provided to the family, and the child's siblings can be monitored with regular eye examinations beginning early in life. As an example, certain types of childhood eye cancers can be caused by a mutation that is inherited. The role that genetics plays in the development of childhood malignancies is only meaningful in a very tiny percentage of cases. There is no evidence of sufficient quality to warrant the implementation of population-based screening programs in children.

Chapter 2

How to reduce the risk of cancer in children

In the United States, there are more than 9000 children are diagnosed with cancer (about 1 in 450). There are many distinct types, but leukemia's, lymphomas, and brain tumours are the most prevalent. There are many other types. Cancer refers to a collection of over one hundred diseases that are brought on when cells in a person's body begin to proliferate in an uncontrolled manner. Cancer is categorized based on the type of cell from which it began (for example, blood, brain, lung), as well as whether or not it has invaded surrounding bodily parts (forming a tumour) or whether or not it has spread to other organs (metastasis). It's possible that I oversimplified things there, but hopefully, you get the point.

It is impossible for you to alter the fact that your DNA will be passed down to your offspring, increasing their likelihood of developing cancer. However, factors such as lifestyle and environment also contribute to their risk, and you have some control in these areas.

This impact takes into account not only the things that your children are exposed to when they are younger but also the examples that they see you set with your behavior and the routines that you establish for them that they will carry with them into their adult lives. They will benefit from the guidance they receive while they are young throughout their life.

How to reduce your child's risk of developing cancer by the following steps:

1. To begin, the most obvious recommendation is that you should not use tobacco and should not permit anybody else to smoke near your children. I am aware that this is easier said than done, yet it is estimated that tobacco use is the cause of four out of every five malignancies. Tobacco's carcinogens cause DNA damage, contributing to an increased risk of developing 14 distinct types of cancer, including lung, some types of leukemia, voice box, throat, liver, and kidney cancers. Being exposed to secondhand smoke raises the risk of cancer by 25%. In contrast to the smoke exhaled, the smoke produced by the burning end of a cigarette contains three times as much carbon monoxide, ten times as many nitrosamines, and hundreds of times as much ammonia. Add to this the fact that if you smoke, your child has a 25 times greater

probability of developing a daily addiction to smoking, which raises their risk even further. Just don't. No justification will do.

2. Another common advice is to shield children from the sun to reduce their risk of developing skin cancer. Always reapply sunscreen, preferably with an SPF of at least 15, throughout the day. Seek shade during busy hours. Put a cap on their head that shadows their face and a pair of sunglasses on their nose, and they will be protected from the sun.

3. Provide them with a nutritious diet that is fiber abundant in fresh fruits and vegetables. Steer clear of processed foods and excessive amounts of salt and red meat. If you eat well, your body will be better able to get rid of cancer-causing chemicals, prevent and repair DNA damage, and prevent other cancer-causing substances from forming. Cancers of the breast, mouth, esophagus and gastrointestinal tract have all been related to an unhealthy diet.

4. Encourage exercising. The hormones like estrogen and insulin, which have been related to cancer, become more stable when one exercises. Cancers of the breast, bowel, and uterus are less likely to occur in those who lead active lifestyles.

5. Ensure that they maintain a healthy weight for their body. Hormones are produced by fatty tissue, which plays a role in determining how cells grow. The abnormal

proliferation of cells is the fundamental cause of cancer. Several malignancies, including those of the breast, esophagus, and intestine, as well as the liver, kidney, pancreas, and uterus, have been related to obesity.

6. Restrict the amount of chemical exposure they get. Recent research has indicated that children's exposure to pesticides within their homes can increase their risk of developing leukemia by 47%. Because cancer-causing chemicals like arsenic, benzene, and asbestos are still used in industry, it is important to be aware of the substances to which you may be exposed while working, to wear the right safety gear, and to avoid bringing any poisons into your home on your clothing. Check the goods you use at home to see if they have any special directions for use (such as "do they need to be used in a well-ventilated area?") and if they have any unusual ingredients. You can research potentially hazardous components of common household goods. Household chemicals such as cleaners, paints, degreasers, and strippers should be kept locked away and stored at a high location for safety.

7. In the category of "set a good example for others," try to minimize the amount of alcohol you drink. Drinking alcohol raises the quantities of substances in your body that can cause cancer and mess with your hormone balances. Additionally, it heightens the harmful effects of cigarette use. Consuming alcohol raises the likelihood that

a person may get breast, mouth, throat, and intestines cancer.

8. Take precautions to prevent some types of illnesses. Because infection can cause persistent inflammation and depress the immune system, it can also increase cancer risk. Your child's risk of contracting hepatitis B increases, so ensure they get vaccinated against it and instruct them to abstain from injecting drugs and engaging in risky sexual behavior. Take precautions with tattoos because the chance of contracting Hepatitis C is also increased, and 41% of that risk comes from tattoos. Helicobacter pylori raise the possibility of developing cancer, and clinicians test for its presence in patients with reflux disease, gastritis, and ulcers. The Human Papillomavirus accomplishes its goals by prompting fast cell division (hence the appearance of a wart). Every year, we lose 4,000 women to cancer that may be prevented, called cervical cancer, and the number of mouth cancers caused by HPV is skyrocketing at an alarming rate.

Cancer risk factors appear to have the greatest impact on a baby while it is still developing inside of its mother's womb, as well as during adolescence when a person's body is rapidly developing and changing; consequently, these are the stages of life during which a parent can unquestionably affect the prevention of cancer. Your child's risk of developing cancer is drastically reduced if you model a healthy lifestyle and encourage them to make healthy food choices. Protect children against sunburns and pollutants that can cause cancer, make sure they get the vaccines they need, teach them healthy behaviors, and set a good example for them. There is no downside to maintaining a nutritious diet, regular exercise routine, and minimizing their exposure to contaminants, all of which may improve the likelihood that they will be around for a while.

Chapter 3

Symptoms that could point to childhood leukemia

Most of the time, leukemia is not the root cause of many of the symptoms associated with childhood leukemia. These symptoms can have other origins. However, suppose your child exhibits any of these symptoms. In that case, you must take them to a medical professional as soon as possible so that the underlying reason can be identified and treated, if necessary.

Leukemia manifests itself in the bone marrow, where healthy new blood cells produce. In many cases, the symptoms of leukemia are brought on by issues originating in the bone marrow. Normal blood cells can be crowded out of the bone marrow while leukemia cells accumulate. Consequently, a child's typical levels of red blood cells, white blood cells, and blood platelets may be depleted. These deficiencies will appear on blood testing, but they may also manifest in other ways. There is a possibility that leukemia cells will spread to other parts of the body, which may also result in symptoms.

The following are symptoms of low red blood cell counts, sometimes known as anemia: Every cell in the body relies on oxygen delivered to it by red blood cells. Having fewer red blood cells in the body can result in several symptoms, including feeling weary (fatigue), feeling weak, chilly, dizzy or lightheaded, shortness of breath, a pale complexion, and feeling lightheaded.

Signs that there is a deficiency in normal white blood cells include the following: The immune system relies on white blood cells to fight off infectious agents. It is common for children with leukemia to have high white blood cell counts; however, most of these cells are leukemia cells, which do not provide adequate protection against infection, and there are not enough normal white blood cells. This can result in the following: • Infections, which can manifest themselves as a result of a deficiency in normal white blood cells. Children with leukemia are at an increased risk of contracting infections, some of which may not go away or acquire infections one after the other.

• High temperature is frequently the most noticeable symptom of an illness. However, there is a possibility that some children will have a fever even if they do not have an infection.

Symptoms of decreased platelet counts in the blood include the following: Platelets work to clot and stop bleeding in healthy individuals. A low platelet count might result in the following symptoms: • Bruising and bleeding more easily

• Frequent or severe nosebleeds

• Bleeding gums

Pain in the bones or joints: This pain is brought on by accumulated leukemia cells close to the bone's surface or within the joint.

Inflammation in the abdominal cavity (the belly): It is possible for leukemia cells to concentrate in the liver and spleen, which then causes those organs to enlarge. This could be experienced as a feeling of fullness or an expansion of the belly. The lower ribs typically hide these organs, but when they are enlarged, a doctor can frequently feel them through the rib cage.

A decrease in appetite and a loss of weight: When the spleen and/or liver become sufficiently large, they can pressure other organs such as the stomach. This could cause the youngster to feel satisfied after consuming only a tiny amount of food, which could eventually result in the child losing their appetite and weight.

Inflammation of the lymph nodes some forms of leukemia can extend to the lymph nodes, which are generally very small collections of immune cells (about the size of a bean) found throughout the body. Certain areas of the body may have the appearance of lumps under the skin, which are actually swollen lymph nodes (such as on the sides of the neck, in the groin, beneath the arms, or above the collarbone). It's also possible for lymph nodes inside the chest or abdomen to swell up, but this is something that can only be detected by imaging tests like CT or MRI scans.

When a toddler or infant is attempting to fight off an infection, the lymph nodes will frequently swell and become larger. It is much more likely that an infection is the cause of an enlarged lymph node in a child rather than leukemia; however, the lymph node should still be evaluated by a doctor and properly monitored.

Coughing and breathing problems can be symptoms of certain types of leukemia, which can damage tissues in the center of the chest, such as the lymph nodes and the thymus (a small organ in front of the trachea, the breathing tube that leads to the lungs). Coughing and problems breathing can be caused when the trachea is compressed due to pressure from an enlarged thymus or lymph nodes in the chest.

In certain instances, when the white blood cell count is extremely high, leukemia cells can accumulate in the small blood arteries of the lungs, which can also cause difficulty breathing. This is one of the symptoms of this condition.

Face and arm swelling: an enlarged thymus may push on the superior vena cava (SVC), which is a big vein that conducts blood returning from the arms and head to the heart. If this occurs, the patient may have swelling of the face and arms. This might result in the blood "pooling" in the veins of the body. This condition is referred to as SVC syndrome. It is possible for there to be swelling in the face, neck, arms, and upper chest as a result of it (sometimes with a bluish-red skin color). If the condition affects the brain, further symptoms may include headaches, dizziness, and even a shift in one's state of consciousness. Because the SVC condition poses a potential risk to one's life, prompt medical attention is required.

A tiny percentage of children are diagnosed with leukemia which had already progressed to the brain and spinal cord when it was first discovered. This type of leukemia is characterized by symptoms such as headaches, convulsions, and vomiting. This can result in symptoms such as headaches, difficulty concentrating, weakness, seizures, vomiting, issues maintaining balance, and blurred vision.

Rashes or issues with the gums: It is possible for leukemia cells to spread to the gums of children who have acute myeloid leukemia (AML), which can result in swelling, discomfort, and gushing.

Once AML has spread to the skin, it can create spots that are small and dark and appear to be rashes that are more common. Chloromas and granulocytic sarcomas are both terms that refer to the same thing: a collection of AML cells that can be found either under the skin or in other places of the body.

Extreme exhaustion and a lack of strength: Extreme fatigue, weakness, and slurred speech are symptoms of AML that are uncommon but highly significant consequences of the disease. When very high numbers of leukemia cells thicken the blood and limit circulation via the small blood arteries of the brain, this can be a potential outcome.

Once more, the majority of the aforementioned symptoms are more likely to be brought on by something other than leukemia. However, it is essential to get these symptoms examined by a medical professional in order to identify the underlying reason and, if necessary, receive treatment for it.

Leukemia in Children Displays These Symptoms

A trip to the physician is frequently prompted by the presence of leukemia symptoms. This is a positive development since it suggests that the illness may be detected earlier than it otherwise would have been. More effective treatment might be possible with an early diagnosis.

When leukemia cells crowd out normal cells, it can cause a number of signs and symptoms that are associated with juvenile leukemia.

The following are examples of common symptoms: tiredness or pale complexion; infections; fever; easy bleeding or bruising; extreme fatigue or weakness; shortness of breath; coughing

Other possible symptoms include the following:

• Pain in the bones or joints

• Swelling in the groin, sides of the neck, cheeks, arms, underarms, or belly

• Swelling above the collarbone

• Vomiting

• Rashes

• Gum difficulties

• Loss of appetite or weight loss

• Headaches, seizures, balance problems, or altered eyesight

• Loss of appetite or weight loss

The Process of Diagnosing Leukemia in Children

In order to arrive at a diagnosis of juvenile leukemia, the attending physician will do a comprehensive physical examination and review the patient's medical history. Diagnostic procedures are utilized in order to determine the subtype of juvenile leukemia that is present.

The initial testing may consist of:

• Blood tests to determine the number of blood cells and observe how they look;

• Bone marrow aspiration and biopsy, which are often obtained from the pelvic bone to confirm a diagnosis of leukemia; and

• Other tests as determined by the physician.

• A lumbar puncture, often known as a spinal tap, examines the fluid that surrounds the brain and spinal cord in order to look for signs of the spread of leukemia cells.

Under a microscope, a pathologist examines the cells that were taken from the blood tests. This expert examines samples taken from bone marrow to determine the total number of blood-forming cells as well as fat cells.

There are a variety of other tests that could be performed to assist in determining the subtype of leukemia that your child may have. These tests also assist physicians in determining the likelihood that leukemia will respond favorably to treatment.

In order to monitor how well your kid is responding to treatment, these tests might be performed again later.

The Treatments Available for Leukemia in Children

Discuss the best alternatives for your child in an open discussion with the doctor treating them for cancer and other team members. The treatment is determined primarily by the subtype of leukemia, in addition to other factors.

Over time, there has been a general upward trend in the percentage of patients who survive their childhood leukemia. In addition, treatment at specialist facilities for children and adolescents offers the benefits of individualized attention. Malignancies that occur in children typically respond better to treatment than cancers that occur in adults, and the bodies of children typically tolerate treatment better.

Sometimes a child with cancer needs treatment to address disease problems before beginning treatment for the cancer itself. Alterations in blood cells, for instance, can trigger infections or severe bleeding, and they can also reduce the amount of oxygen that reaches the tissues of the body. Antibiotics, blood transfusions, and other anti-infective methods are among the potential treatments for this infection.

The most common form of treatment for children is chemotherapy. Leukemia. Your child may take the anticancer medication orally, have it injected into a vein, or have it infused into the spinal fluid. To keep leukemia Repeated cycles over the course of two or three years may be necessary in order to prevent the disease from reappearing.

Additionally, targeted therapy is utilized on occasion. This treatment takes a more targeted approach than traditional chemotherapy by focusing on particular aspects of cancer cells. Beneficial for a number of different types of children leukemia, the adverse effects of targeted therapies are typically less severe.

Radiation therapy is one option among many others when it comes to treatments. High-energy radiation is used in this method to kill cancer cells and shrink tumors. It can also help prevent or treat the spread of leukemia to other parts of the body. Surgery is rarely an option to treat childhood leukemia.

If standard treatment is likely to be less effective, a stem cell transplant may be the best option. It involves a transplant of blood-forming stem cells after whole-body radiation combined with high-dose chemotherapy happens first to destroy the child's bone marrow.

The FDA has approved a type of gene therapy for children and young adults up to age 25 whose B-cell ALL doesn't get better with other treatments. Scientists are working on a version of this treatment for people over 25 and for other kinds of cancer.

The CAR T-cell therapy employs part of the patient's own T cells from the immune system in order to treat the patient's malignancy. The cells are removed from your blood and then modified by the addition of new genes by a medical professional. The newly developed T cells are more capable of locating and eliminating cancer cells. Although childhood cancer is rare, leukemia is the most common form. The cause of leukemia is unknown, but we do know that it does not spread to other people ("catching"). It is not believed to be inherited in most cases (inherited from your parents).According to the findings of recent studies, there is a connection between exposure to certain environmental factors and the development of this particular form of cancer.

Leukemia is a type of cancer that occurs in the bone marrow. The tissue that may be found inside of many of the bones in the body is referred to as bone marrow. Blood is produced in the bone marrow of animals. With leukemia, in the bone marrow, there is an excessive proliferation of immature cells that are referred to as blasts or "leukemic cells." Because of the high volume of blasts that are produced, the gaps in the bone marrow become congested. The production of normal blood cells—including red cells, white cells, and platelets—is inhibited as a result of the congestion.

As a result of the disease process, the blood has a decreased number of normal blood cells and an increased number of leukemic cells.

There are primarily two different kinds of childhood leukemia:

• Acute lymphocytic leukemia (ALL) – this type accounts for 80 percent of all leukemia in children.

• Acute myeloid leukemia (AML) is the category that makes up twenty percent of the total.

Signs and Symptoms of Leukemia The symptoms of leukemia are caused by a reduction in the number of normal blood cells leukemia.

• When the amount of red blood cells is small, a child is anemic and may become lean, sluggish and prone to exhaustion.

- If the child has a low white cell count, they have an increased risk of contracting infections and may experience fever as a result.
- The kid may experience discomfort in the bones;
- The child's spleen and belly may be swollen and sore to the touch;
- The child may have bleeding difficulties, such as nosebleeds and increased bruising, when the amount of platelets in the blood is low.

Diagnosis

- The diagnosis of leukemia bone marrow aspirate and perhaps a bone marrow biopsy are both required before a diagnosis may be determined. A pathologist uses a microscope to analyze the tissue of the bone marrow in a patient. The doctor will be able to tell what kind of cancer the patient has based on the findings of this treatment leukemia the child has.
- A lumbar spine test (LP) or spinal tap, of which a little amount (1/2 to 1 teaspoon) of spinal fluid is removed for examination, is also done. This shows if leukemia involves the central nervous system.

Treatment

- Treatment of acute leukemia involves the use of chemotherapy and possibly radiation therapy. Both radiation and chemotherapy destroy the leukemia cells that crowd out normal blood cells. Some treatments are done on an outpatient basis.

• With prompt treatment, a cure or long, disease-free response is possible for many children with ALL or AML. If acute leukemia are not healed,

• A full remission is obtained when there are no identifiable leukemic cells in the bone marrow. • All of these forms of leukemia are lethal within a matter of weeks or months.

• A transplant of bone marrow is another potential course of treatment that could be considered. If your kid may be a candidate for a bone marrow transplant; the physicians and nurses caring for them will provide you with additional information.

• During your child's therapy for some conditions, he or she may need to get blood transfusions leukemia.

• Treatment usually takes about two years for girls and three years for boys.

Few is known about the causes of childhood leukemia. Little things have been shown NOT to cause leukemia. Leukemia is not the result of consuming food or drink. It is not due to the air that we breathe in any way. There is no connection to electrical lines or mobile phones in any way. You won't be able to catch leukemia.

Most of the time, leukemia is not genetic. This means it does not come from your parents. Having a brother or sister with leukemia can very rarely increase your risk of having leukemia.

The immune system is part of the body that fights infection. The immune system helps our bodies fight cancer. Scientists believe that changes in the immune system may increase the risk of developing leukemia. Children who get chemotherapy or radiation to treat other types of cancer have an increased risk of developing leukemia later on.

Children with certain genetic conditions, such as Down syndrome or Li-Fraumeni syndrome, are at increased risk of developing leukemia.

Chapter 4

The signs and symptoms of childhood cancer

Many malignancies in children are discovered at an early stage, either by the child's doctor or by the parents or other family members. On the other hand, it is not always easy to spot cancer in its early stages in youngsters because the symptoms are sometimes similar to those produced by far more common illnesses or accidents. Children frequently experience illnesses or have bumps or bruises, which might hide the early symptoms of diseases such as cancer. It is not common for children to develop cancer, but it is important to have children check by doctor if they have unusual signs or symptoms that do not go away. Some of these signs and symptoms include:
• An unusual lump or swelling
• Unexplained paleness and loss of energy
• Easy bruising or bleeding

- An ongoing pain in one area of the body
- Limping
- Unexplained fever or illness that does not go away
- Frequent headaches, often with vomiting.

The majority of these symptoms are considerably more likely to be brought on by anything other than cancer, like an injury or an infection. However, if your child displays any of these symptoms, it is imperative that you take them to a medical professional immediately so that the root cause can be identified and, if necessary, treated.

There may be additional symptoms, but they may vary according to the type of cancer. You can find additional information about the symptoms that are common for particular types of children's cancer.

Cancer in children can be challenging to diagnose. The following list of signs and symptoms, many of which are comparable to other illnesses that are common in children, may be experienced by children who are afflicted with cancer. Changes that you can sense occurring in your body are referred to as symptoms. Changes in something that can be measured, like your blood pressure or the results of a lab test, can serve as indicators of a potential health problem. Individually or in combination, symptoms and indicators can serve to characterize a medical situation. Sometimes, children who have cancer will display none of the symptoms and signs that are listed here. Alternatively, a health problem that is not cancer could be the root cause of a symptom or indicator of the disease.

• A persistent and mysterious loss of weight

• Increased swelling or persistent pain in the bones, joints, back, or legs

• Headaches, frequently accompanied by vomiting first thing in the morning

• A lump or tumour, most commonly located in the abdominal region, neck, chest, pelvic, or armpits

• The appearance of excessive bruising, bleeding, or a rash

• Infections that are constant, frequent, or persistent

• A whitish color behind the pupil

• Nausea that persists or vomiting without nausea

• Constant tiredness or noticeable paleness

• Changes in the eye or vision that occur suddenly and persist

• Recurring or persistent fevers of unknown origin

• A whitish color behind the pupil

Please talk with your family physician if you are concerned about any changes in your child's behavior. In addition to asking additional questions, your pediatrician will inquire as to how long and how frequently your child has been exhibiting the symptom(s). This will assist in making a diagnosis, which means determining the cause of the issue.

In the event that cancer is discovered, alleviating symptoms is a crucial component of cancer care as well as a cancer treatment. Symptom management is frequently referred to as "palliative care" and "supporting care." It is often begun soon after the diagnosis is made and is maintained throughout treatment. Be sure to discuss your kid's symptoms, including any new symptoms or changes in their existing symptoms, with the healthcare team that is caring for your child.

Cancer symptoms can often be very difficult to differentiate from those of other children's illnesses. Please keep in mind that cancer is not typically the cause of these symptoms. Make an appointment with your child's physician if they exhibit any of the following symptoms:

• They are unable to urinate or have blood in their urine;
• They have an unexplained lump, firmness, or swelling anywhere in their body;
• They have tummy (abdominal) pain or swelling that doesn't go away;
• They have back or bony pain that doesn't go away, or pain that wakes your child up in the night;
• They have seizures (fits) or changes in their behavior and mood;
• They have headaches that don't go away

- Recurrent or inexplicable bruises or a rash of small red or purple patches that cannot be explained;
- Unusual paleness;
- Feeling fatigued all the time;
- Frequent infections or flu-like symptoms
- Alterations in the appearance of the eye or strange eye reflections in photographs
- Feeling short of breath
- being sick for no apparent reason
- Inexplicable vomiting (being sick)
- Unexplained high temperature (fever) or sweating
- Feeling sick for no apparent reason

Despite the fact that cancer in children is extremely uncommon, it is the second leading cause of death among children in developed countries. It frequently manifests with nonspecific symptoms that are similar to those of benign illnesses, which results in delays in the diagnosis and the commencement of treatment which is suitable. When treating children who have concerning or ongoing signs and symptoms, primary care providers should have a higher index of suspicion and investigate the possibility of cancer. Symptoms such as unexplained and prolonged pallor, malaise, fever, anorexia, weight loss, lymphadenopathy, hemorrhagic diathesis, and hepatosplenomegaly are all red flag indicators that could indicate leukemia or lymphoma. It is important to be wary of tumours of the central nervous system if you have just begun experiencing or continue to have morning headaches that are accompanied by vomiting, neurologic symptoms, or back pain. Abdominal, soft tissue and bone tumours can be suspected when there are palpable lumps in the belly or soft tissues and when the kid experiences recurrent bone discomfort that wakes them up. Leukokoria is a red indicator for retinoblastoma. Endocrinal and germ cell tumours could be the cause of endocrine symptoms such as growth stops, diabetes insipid us, and premature or delayed puberty. Rare par neoplastic signs such as opsoclonus-myoclonus syndrome, rheumatic symptoms, or hypertension may be associated with neuroblastoma, leukemia, or Wilms tumour, respectively. Conditions that are associated with higher risk of childhood cancer include immunodeficiency syndromes and previous malignancies. Additionally, increased suspicion is warranted for certain genetic conditions and familial cancer syndromes such as Down syndrome, Li-Fraumeni syndrome, hemihypertrophy, neurofibromatosis, and retinoblastoma.

When should you make an appointment to visit a doctor about your symptoms?

It is common for the early symptoms of cancer in children to be identical to the symptoms of other, less dangerous disorders; as a result, it is easy to overlook them. For example, you might not immediately connect your child's exhaustion or the pain in their joints to leukemia, which is the most prevalent form of cancer found in youngsters. It's possible that you'll brush it off as normal teenage angst. But if you sense something is off with your child, or if they tell you about a new and persistent symptom they're feeling, it's always a good idea to check in with your child's pediatrician, especially if the illness seems to be getting worse over time.

Contact your child's primary care physician as soon as possible if you observe any of the following symptoms in your child:

• Unusual mass or swelling
• Unexplained paleness or worsening rash
• Loss of energy for no apparent reason
• Unusual behavior or movements
• Sudden tendency to bruise or bleed easily
• Lasting pain in any part of the body
• Unexplained fever that doesn't go away
• Frequent headaches, often with vomiting
• Sudden eye or vision changes
• Unexpected, rapid weight loss

When children exhibit symptoms of cancer that linger for a while or cause significant pain or discomfort, doctors may offer certain tests to rule out other causes before looking for cancer. This is done to ensure that the symptoms are not caused by something other than cancer. The diagnostic processes and testing for cancer vary greatly based on the suspected cancer type. The tests could consist of a physical examination, blood test, X-ray, ultrasound, CT scan, MRI, PET/CT scan, CT scan, or biopsy.

Chapter 5

Diagnosis of cancer in children

In order to detect or diagnose cancer, doctors perform a variety of tests. They also perform tests to determine whether or not the cancer has progressed to another section of the body from the location where it initially manifested itself. The term "metastasis" refers to the spread of cancer throughout the body. Tests are another option for doctors to investigate potential remedies might work best.

A biopsy is the only way for the doctor to know for certain, regardless of the type of cancer, whether or not a particular location of the body has cancer. During a biopsy, the physician removes a sample of tissue from the tumour tissue sample for examination in a scientific setting. In the event that the physician is unable to perform a biopsy, he or she may recommend other diagnostic procedure to help diagnose.

When selecting a diagnostic test for your child, the doctor may take into consideration the following factors:

The form of cancer that is possibly present

The symptoms and indicators that your kid is experiencing

The age of your child as well as his or her overall health

According to the findings of past diagnostic procedures

Only some tests described here will be used for some people. It is important to have tests done in a pediatric specialist center where tests can be supervised by pediatric specialists. These are medical professionals who specialize in diagnosing and treating younger patients. In addition a physical examination, the following tests may be used to diagnose childhood cancer:

·   **Blood tests.** Routine blood tests measure the number of different types of cells in a person's blood. Levels of certain cells that are too high or too low can indicate the presence of certain types of cancer.

·   **Biopsy.** A biopsy removes little size of a tissue sample that will be examined under a microscope. The only test that can detect cancer is a biopsy. Definitively diagnose cancer, with a few exceptions for certain types of brain tumors. Other procedures may raise the possibility of cancer being present tumours. A biopsy can be guided by imaging tests (such as computed tomography (CT) or magnetic resonance imaging (MRI) scan; see below) to make the procedure accurate and precise. The type of biopsy depends on the tumor's location and part of the body involved. A pathologist will conduct an examination on the tissue sample that was taken during the biopsy. A physician who specializes in the interpretation of laboratory tests and the evaluation of cells, tissues, and organs in order to identify disease is called a pathologist.

· **Bone marrow aspiration and biopsy.** These two procedures are similar and often done simultaneously to examine the bone marrow, which is the spongy, fatty tissue found inside larger bones. The marrow of bones can be found in both a solid and a liquid state. An aspiration of the bone marrow involves the removal of a sample of the fluid using a needle. A needle is used to extract a small sample of solid tissue from the bone marrow during a procedure known as a biopsy.
A pathologist, in that case studies the samples in a lab. The pelvic bone, which can be found close to the hip, is frequently used as the extraction point for bone marrow as well as the biopsy site. In most cases, patients receive a specific class of drug known as anesthesia beforehand to numb the area. Anesthesia is the medication that blocks the awareness of pain.

· Lumbar puncture (spinal tap). A needle is used to extract a sample of fluid from the patient's lumbar region during a procedure known as a lumbar puncture. Cerebral spinal fluid (CSF) to look for cancer cells or tumour markers. Tumour markers are substances found in higher than normal amounts in the blood, urine, or body tissues of people with certain kinds of cancer. The cerebrospinal fluid, often known as CSF, is the fluid that circulates around the brain and the spinal cord. Patients are often given an anesthetic to numb the lower back before the procedure or other medications to calm or relax your child (sedation).

·   **Ultrasound** An ultrasound produces a picture of the interior organs by using sound waves to create the image. Patients are usually awake during an ultrasound.

· Computed tomography scan, often known as a CAT or CT scan. A computed tomography (CT) scan uses multiple projections of x-rays to produce internal images of the patient's body. After that, a computer will merge all of these images into a comprehensive, three-dimensional picture that will highlight any anomalies or tumours. In addition to this, a CT scan can also be utilized to measure the tumour's size. Before the scan, it is not uncommon for a specialized dye known as a contrast medium to be administered in order to improve the image's level of detail. This dye can either be administered intravenously by injecting it into a patient's vein or orally in the form of a pill or liquid to be swallowed. When possible, it is best to have this test done in a pediatric specialist center where it can be supervised by pediatric radiologists. These centers are aware of the potential risks of radiation exposure from a CT scan.

· Magnetic resonance imaging (MRI). The magnetic resonance imaging (MRI) technique produces more comprehensive images of the human body than x-rays do. MRI can also be used to measure the tumour's size. In order to produce a more distinct image, a contrast medium, which is a specialized dye, is applied before the scan. It is possible to administer this dye to a patient in the form of an injection into a vein, as well as in the form of a pill or liquid to be swallowed. Positron emission tomography (PET) or PET-CT scan. The combination of a PET scan and a CT scan is typically referred to as a PET-CT scan. On the other hand, your physician might casually refer to this test as a PET scan in casual conversation. A PET scan is a type of imaging test that can be used to generate images of the organs and tissues found inside the body. A very minute quantity of a radioactive sugar compound is administered intravenously to the patient. The cells that consume the most energy are the ones that take in this sugar molecule. Because cancer has a propensity to make active use of energy, it is able to absorb a greater quantity of the radioactive chemical. On the other hand, the amount of radiation contained in the chemical is insufficient to be dangerous patients.

Following this, a scanner will identify this chemical in order to make images of the internal organs.

Scans or radioisotope studies. In these procedures, a material with a small amount of radioactive substance (called a tracer) is injected into the body and then followed with a special camera or x-ray to see where the material goes. These studies can find abnormalities in the liver, brain, bones, kidneys, and other organs.

A person needs to go through a series of tests in order to determine whether or not they have cancer, or whether or not cancer symptoms are being caused by anything else (such an infection, for example). When a person's condition changes, or when a sample of tissue or fluid gathered from them does not match expectations, more testing may be required. Is not of good quality, or in the event that an anomalous test result needs to have its validity verified.

In order to properly direct treatment, a precise diagnosis is required. The following tests are frequently included in a diagnostic battery for cancer, in addition to a comprehensive medical history and physical examination: Blood count taken in its entirety (CBC).

When drawing blood from a vein in the hand or arm, a very thin needle is typically utilized.

This blood test will determine the size, quantity, and maturity of certain blood cells that are present in your blood.

Unusual cells could be an early indicator of malignancy. Alterations in the typical amount of cells, their size, and the stage at which they mature can all be indicators of cancer.

Aspiration of the bone marrow, a biopsy, or both may be performed.

During this treatment, either a little amount of fluid from the bone marrow (known as an aspiration) or solid bone marrow tissue will be removed (called a core biopsy).

This is often performed from the posterior aspect of the hip bones.

The number of aberrant cells, their size, and their level of development are assessed using the samples that have been removed.

Spinal tap (lumbar puncture).

This operation is carried out to examine the fluid that surrounds the spine and brain for signs of infection or pressure, as well as to look for any abnormal cells that may be present.

In order to access the spinal canal, a tiny needle is inserted between the bones of the lower back.

This refers to the region that encompasses the spinal cord.

After that, the pressure in the brain as well as the spinal canal can be monitored.

To determine if there is an infection or some other issue, a small sample of cerebral spinal fluid (also known as CSF) can be extracted and sent away for testing.

The brain and spinal cord are both bathed and cushioned by a fluid called cerebrospinal fluid (CSF).

Lymph angiogram (LAG).

The purpose of this imaging examination is to search for cancerous cells as well as abnormalities in the lymph veins and tissues (such as lymph nodes).

An injection of a dye is given to a lymph vessel.

After that, images are performed to demonstrate the path that the dye takes through the lymphatic system.

Ultrasound (sonographer).

This is an imaging test that utilizes sound waves and a computer in order to generate images of the organs, tissues, and blood arteries within the body.

It is performed by moving a tiny wand over the skin of the area of the body that is to be examined.

- It is possible to observe, via ultrasound, the functioning of internal organs as well as the movement of blood through blood vessels. Tumours in the stomach, liver, and kidneys can often be seen with an ultrasound.

Tumour biopsy. A biopsy requires the removal of a very small sample of tissue from the tumour been validated in a laboratory. This could be accomplished with the use of a needle or through surgical procedures. Because they provide the most accurate examination and testing of tissue, biopsies are frequently required in order to arrive at a diagnosis.

- Bone scans. A radioactive dye is injected into the bloodstream through a vein, and the bone then takes up the radioactive dye. After that, scans will indicate where the dye has accumulated. It's possible that these "hotspots" are tumours or other bone abnormalities.
- **X-rays.** These tests use beams of radiation to make images of tissues, bones, and organs on film. X-rays may be taken of any part of the body to look for a tumour.

CT scan.

- In this type of imaging test, X-rays and a computer work together to create extremely detailed images of the inside of the body. CT scan shows details of the bones, muscles, fat, and organs. The person lies on a thin table that slides through a ring-shaped scanner to do this test.

- **PET-CT (positron emission tomography and CT scans).** A radioactive sugar is put in the blood before this test. It collects in areas of active cells. Then the CT scan makes detailed pictures of tissues and organs, while the PET scan shows abnormal cell activity. A complete image is provided by combining these tests. The person lies on a narrow table that slowly moves through a series of ring-shaped scanners to do this test,

- **MRI.** An MRI uses large magnets, radio frequencies, and a computer to make detailed images of organs and structures inside the body. This test doesn't use X-rays. But the table the person lies on slides through a long, thin, tube-like scanner. Some people have trouble being inside the narrow scanner.

- **Blood tests.** Blood tests are used to look at a person's electrolytes, liver function, kidney function, presence of infection, tumour markers (chemicals released by a tumour), or genetic testing. Genetic counselling may be advised for families that are found or believed to have an inherited risk of cancer. A needle is used to get the blood for this test from a vein in the arm or hand.

- **Surgery.** Surgery may be needed to do a biopsy, remove tumours, remove organs affected by the disease, and look for tumours that may not be found with imaging tests. There are many kinds of surgery that can be done.

www.ingramcontent.com/pod-product-compliance
Lightning Source LLC
Chambersburg PA
CBHW061614250726
48653CB00014B/2877